Lose Up Pounds with Keto Diet

Lose Pounds with Keto Recipes Easily

By Alan Williams

Table Of Content

SEAFOOD RECIPES

BUTTERED COD

Ingredients

- 1 ½ lbs of cod fillets

- 6 Tbsp unsalted butter, sliced

- seasoning

- ¼ tsp garlic powder

- ½ tsp table salt

- ¼ tsp ground pepper

- ¾ tsp ground pepper

- Some slices of lemon

- Herbs, parsley or coriander

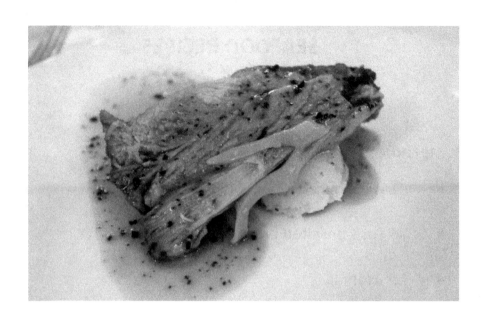

Instructions

How to make a cod with butter in a pan

1.   Mix herbal ingredients in a small bowl.

2.   Cut the cord into small pieces, if you wish. Season with the herbs.

3.   Heat 2 Tbsp butter in a large skillet over medium-high heat. As soon as the butter melts, add the cod to the pan. Cook 2 min

4.   Lower the heat to medium. Turn the cod over, cover with the remaining butter, and cook another 3-4 min

5.   The butter melts completely, and the fish boils. (Do not overfish the cod, it will soften and collapse completely).

6.   Sprinkle the cod with fresh lemon juice. Cover with fresh herbs if desired.

Prep time:5 min; Servings: 4

Macros: Cal 294 Lipids 18g28% Saturated fat 11g69% Cholesterol 118 mg 39% Sodium 385 mg 17% Potassium

712 mg 20% 30 g of 60% protein Vitamin A 815IU16%
Vitamin C 1.7 mg2% Calcium 32mg3% Iron 0.7 mg4%

SEMOLINA WITH LOADED CAULIFLOWER

RICE

Ingredients

- 2 bags of 12 oz chopped cauliflower

- 2 lbs of shrimp (shelled and deveined)

- 1 block of 8 oz strong cheddar cheese

- 1 block of 8 g of Pepper Jack cheese

- 1 cup thick whipped cream

- 4 Tbsp salted butter

- 3/4 cup white mushrooms

- 6 thick strips of bacon

- 1 lemon (juiced)

- 1 bunch of chopped green onions

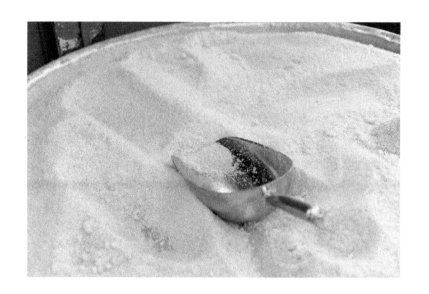

Instructions

1.   Cook the bacon.

2.   Rinse the shrimp.

3.   Rinse and cut the mushrooms.

4.   Add grated cheeses.

5.   Prepare cauliflower rice

6.   Place cauliflower cheese in a large medium saucepan over low heat. Add the thick cream.

7.   In another pan, saute shrimp, mushrooms, lemon juice, butter, and about 2 Tbsp bacon until shrimp is golden brown.

8.   Combine cauliflower rice + shrimp and cover with green onions

Servings: 6; Prep time:15 min

SHRIMP AND SPINACH CREAM SAUCE

Ingredients

- 2 Tbsp unsalted butter

- 1 lb of shrimp - peeled, deveined

- 1 tsp onion powder

- 1 tsp garlic powder

- ½ cup thick cream

- ½ cup cream cheese - diced

- ½ cup water

- 6-8 cups fresh spinach

- Salt pepper

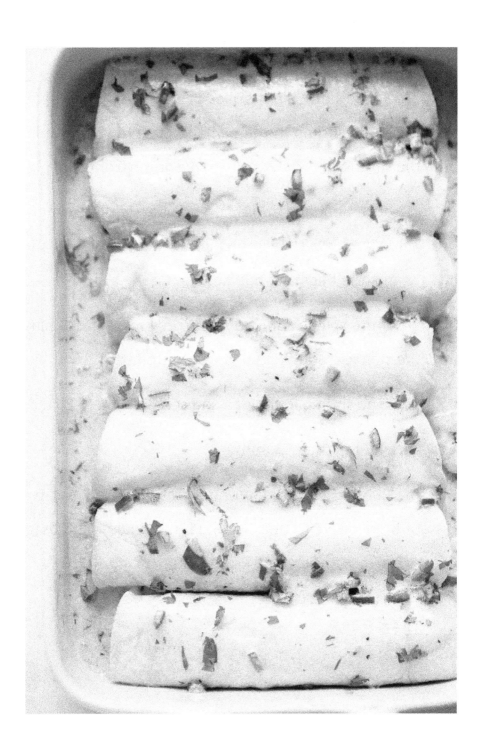

Instructions

1.   Melt the butter in a skillet over medium-high heat skillet. Put the shrimp in the pan and cook for 2 to 4 min until the shrimp are cooked. Remove shrimp from pan.

2.   Reduce heat and add onion powder, garlic powder, heavy cream, cream cheese, and water. Beat until smooth, and the mixture begins to bubble.

3.   Add the spinach and cook, stirring, for 8 to 10 min, until the spinach fades. Salt and pepper to taste.

4.   Put the shrimp in the pan and serve.

Servings: 4; Prep time:15 min

Macros: Cal 476 Fat 30g Saturated fat 17g Trans fat 0g Unsaturated fat 10g Cholesterol 317mg Sodium 1460mg Carbs 18g Fiber 8g Sugar 4g Protein 39g

KETO FRIT FISH

Ingredients

- 1 lb of whitefish, tilapia, or saithe cod works excellent!

- 3/4 cup almond flour

- Salt and pepper

- 2-3 tsp Tony Chachere creole herbs

- 2 beaten eggs

- Frying oil I used about ½ cup beef tallow

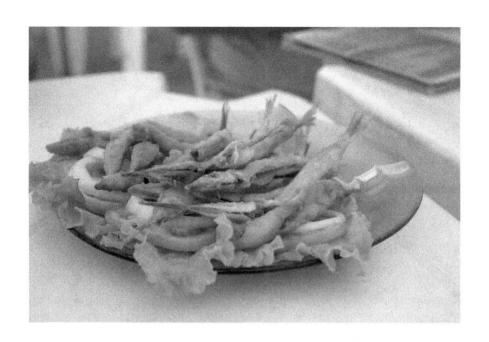

Instructions

1.   Heat the oil over medium heat in a heavy frying pan. If you have an electric pot, set it to 375 F

2.   Place the beaten eggs on a rectangular plate. Then mix the almond flour and Tony's flour (or other spices) and place it in a shallow dish or dish to soak the fish.

3.   Dry the fish with a paper towel, season both sides with salt and pepper in the egg, and cover both sides with the almond flour mixture while stirring to remove the excess.

4.   Place the fish in the hot oil in the pan. Bake 2 to 4 minutes per side.

Prep time:10 min; Servings: 4

Macros: Cal 344 | Carbs 4 g | Protein 25 g | Lipids: 25 g Saturated Fat 1 g | Cholesterol 130 mg | Sodium 92 mg Potassium 498 mg | Fiber 2g | Vitamin A: 165 IU | Vitamin C: 1.2 mg | Calcium: 75 mg Iron: 1.6 mg

HEALTHY SHRIMP WITH ZUCCHINI NOODLES

Ingredients

- 1 Tbsp unsalted butter

- 1 Tbsp olive oil

- 1 finely chopped shallot

- 4 garlic cloves, finely chopped (about 1 ½ Tbsp)

- 1 lb. Giant Raw Shrimp - fresh or frozen and thawed

- 1 tsp kosher salt

- ½ tsp red pepper flakes

- ¼ tsp black pepper

- ¼ cup low sodium chicken broth or white wine

- ½ zest of lemon

- ¼ cup freshly squeezed lemon juice

- 1 ½ lbs of zucchini noodles - about 4 medium-sized zucchini

- ¼ cup chopped fresh parsley leaves

- 2 Tbsp freshly grated Parmesan cheese

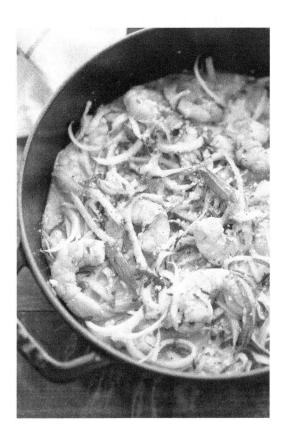

Instructions

1.   Heat the butter and olive oil in a large skillet over medium-high heat. Add the shallot and cook until softened for about 3 min Add garlic and cook for 30 seconds. Add shrimp, salt, pepper flakes, and black pepper. Bake 3 min, until shrimp.

2.   Add chicken broth, lemon zest, and lemon juice. Bring to the boil and cook for 1 minute, until the shrimps are wholly opaque and well prepared.

3.   Add zucchini noodles and parsley. Mix the noodles with the shrimp so that they are covered with garlic and lemon sauce and warm to hot. (Do not overcook. Otherwise, zucchini noodles will become soft). Sprinkle with parsley and parmesan.

Servings: 4; Prep time:15 min

Macros: Cal 224, Fat 9g, Saturated Fat 3g, Cholesterol 295mg, Sodium 1527mg, Potassium 596mg, Carbs 9g, Fiber: 2g, Sugar 5g, Protein 27g, Vitamin A: 520%, Vitamin C

FRIED COD WITH PARMESAN AND HERB

BUTTER

Ingredients

- 3/4 cup freshly grated Parmesan cheese

- ½ lemon (zest, more juice)

- fresh parsley Tbsp (small or finely chopped)

- ½ tsp garlic powder

- 1 ¼ tsp pepper

- Tbsp butter (use a maximum of 5 Tbsp if you want more butter sauce)

- 1 ½ lbs Fresh cod

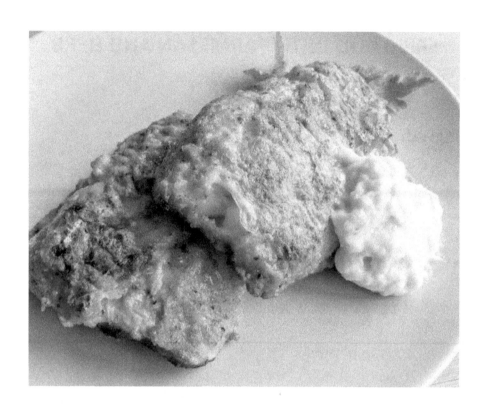

Instructions

1.   Preheat the oven to 400° F. Grease a cooktop rim with spray oil. Place the grated parmesan on the plate and add the garlic powder and pepper.

2.   Wash and dry the lemon. Cut it in half and grate the skin of 1 of the halves. Add it to the cheese mixture.

3.   Rinse the parsley and dry it. Cut it with scissors or cut it before adding it to the cheese mixture. Mix the cheese mix with a fork to mix.

4.   Rinse the fish in cold water and rub your thumbs on the surface to see if there are bones to remove. Dry the fish with paper towels.

5.   Melt the butter in a small saucepan on the stove or in the microwave in a bowl. A place to treadmill from left to right with fish, butter, cheese mixture, and pan.

6.   Use a fork for fishing each other in the butter, then in the cheese mixture, cover both sides, and beat the cod with the fork. Place the coated fish on the dish, cover with an excess of melted butter and bake for 15 min Cod is made when you can easily crumble it with a fork.

7.   Squeeze the lemon juice over the fish.

Prep time:20 min; Servings: 4

Macros: Cal 303 15g fat Saturated fat 8g Cholesterol 112 mg37 Sodium 455 mg Potassium 769 mg Carbs 2G 37 g of protein

LIGHT ROASTED GARLIC SAUCE

Ingredients

- 2 garlic bulbs

- 2 Tbsp olive oil

- 1 Tbsp butter

- 1 ½ cup grated Parmesan cheese

- 6 g of cream cheese

- 1 cup chicken broth

- ½ cup thick cream

- Freshly ground black pepper

Instructions

1.   Cut the top of ¼ garlic bulbs and sprinkle with olive oil.

2.   Make a tent with foil and roast in the oven at 400° F for 1 hour.

3.   Once the garlic is fresh, squeeze the roasted garlic cloves into a bowl and mashed potatoes. Put aside.

4.   Melt the butter in a large saucepan. Add the heavy cream and chicken broth.

5.   Bring to boil and beat regularly.

6.   Add the cheese cream and parmesan cheese. Simmer for 8 to 10 min until thickened.

7.   Season with freshly ground black pepper.

8.   Serve immediately.

Servings: 6; Prep time:10 min

Macros: Cal 338 Total Fat: 30 g Saturated Fat: 15.9 g Cholesterol 79.7 mg Sodium 636 mg Carbs 5.1 g Fiber 0.2 g Sugar 1.7 g Protein 13.7 g

SHRIMP WITH BUTTER

Ingredients

- 1 lb of raw shrimps, shelled and thawed

- 1 Tbsp olive oil

- 4 garlic cloves, finely chopped

- 1 Tbsp lemon juice

- ½ tsp salt

- 3 Tbsp melted butter

- 2 Tbsp fresh parsley, to decorate

- Baked asparagus

- 1 bunch of asparagus

- 1 Tbsp butter

- 1 Tbsp olive oil

Instructions

1. Mix the shelled and thawed shrimp with olive oil, salt, minced garlic, and lemon juice and set aside while cooking the asparagus.

2. Fry asparagus in oil and butter for a few minutes until tender, season with salt and pepper, cover with foil to keep warm, and set aside.

3. Melt the butter in a skillet over medium heat, then add the shrimp and marinade and cook for about 1 to 2 min per side until the shrimp are pink.

4. Serve hot, sprinkled with fresh chopped parsley and asparagus on the side.

Prep time:10 min; Servings: 4

Macros: Total Carbs 5 g Net Carbs 3 g Protein 26 g Cal 304

KETO FISH BOWLS

Ingredients

- 4 frozen cod fillets

- 2 Tbsp melted butter

- 2 Tbsp tacos herbs

- ¼ cup sour cream

- 1 ½ tsp lime juice

- 1 tsp honey

- 1 Tbsp milk

- pinch of salt

- 2 cups of cauliflower with lime and pineapple

- 2 cups sweet and spicy cabbage salad

- 1 sliced avocado

- ¼ cup chopped coriander, to decorate

Instructions

1.   Preheat the oven to 400° F.

2.   Mix the melted butter and taco herbs. Brush the frozen fillets quickly. Bake for 25 min

3.   Mix sour cream, juice lime, honey, milk, and salt.

4.   Fill 4 bowls with ½ cup cauliflower rice, ½ cup cabbage salad, 1 fish fillet, and a few slices of avocado. Sprinkle with cream and coriander.

Prep time:20 min; Servings: 6

CLIMATE KETO

Ingredients

- 5 bacon cut into cubes

- 2 garlic cloves, finely chopped

- ½ diced yellow onions

- ½ tsp dried thyme

- 1 cup unsweetened almond milk

- 1 cup thick cream

- 1 cup chicken broth

- 4 oz cream cheese

- 18 oz drained canned hulls

- 1 bay leaf

- 3 cups of cauliflower flowers

- freshly chopped parsley optional

Instructions

1.   Dutch oven or another heavy-bottomed saucepan over medium heat. Add the chopped bacon and cook until thoroughly cooked. Remove the bacon and save. Keep 3 Tbsp bacon in the pan.

2.   Add onion and garlic. Bake until onion begins to turn transparent (about 2-3 min). Add the thyme and fry for another minute.

3.   Add milk almond, cream, and chicken broth. Mix well and add the cream cheese. Stir until cream cheese melts.

4.   Add bay leaves, hulls, and the cauliflower florets. Bring to a boil, then reduce to medium-low heat, cover, and cook for 5 to 10 min or until cauliflower is tender.

5.   Serve covered with boiled bacon and chopped parsley if necessary.

Prep time:10 min; Servings: 6

Macros: 339 Cal, 25 g oFat, 8 g of Carbs, 2 g oFiber, 19 g of

protein 6 g of net carbs

KETO TUNA CAKES

Ingredients

- 15 g of tuna in spring water 3 boxes of 5 g.

- ⅓ cup fresh herbs, chives, and parsley

- ¼ cup almond flour

- 2 Tbsp low-carb mayonnaise

- 2 tsp lemon zest

- 1 tsp chopped dried onion

- 2 large eggs

- ½ tsp salt

- ¼ tsp ground pepper

- ¼ cup olive oil for frying

Instructions

1.   Drain the tuna well. You should end up with about 280 g of tuna.

2.   In a large bowl, add all ingredients except the oil. Mix well. The mixture will be wet, but it will stay together when you make a ball.

3.   Place a large nonstick skillet over medium-high heat. Place a quarter cup spoon in hot oil and bake for 3-4 min on each side. You should get 8 tuna cookies.

4.   Serve with fresh lemon and a Tbsp low-carb mayonnaise.

Prep time: 10 min; Servings: 4

Macros: Cal 287 | Carbs 3g | Protein 26g | Fat 19 g | Saturated Fat 3g | Cholesterol 146 mg Sodium 641 mg Potassium 277 mg Fiber 1 g | Sugar 1 g | Vitamin A: 635 IU | Vitamin C: 8.8 mg Calcium: 59 mg | Iron: 2.8 mg

CAJUN SAUSAGE AND VEGETABLES

Ingredients

- 1 lb of shrimp, shelled and evaded

- 14 g of sliced pork or chicken sausage

- 2 medium sliced zucchini

- 2 medium-sized yellow carved pumpkins

- ½ bunch of asparagus cut in 3

- 2 chopped red peppers

- Salt and pepper

- 2 Tbsp olive oil

- 2 Tbsp Cajun herbs

Instructions

1.	In a large bowl, add shrimp, sausages, zucchini, yellow squash, asparagus, pepper and salt, and pepper.

Add olive oil and Cajun spices and stir until everything is covered.

2.   Add to a large skillet over medium-high heat. Bake for about 5-7 min

3.   Garnish with fresh parsley.

Prep time: 5 min; Servings: 6

Macros: Cal 260 Lipids 12g18% Saturated fat 2g10% Cholesterol 240 mg 80% Sodium 989 mg 41% Potassium 712 mg 20% Carbs 8g3% 3g12% oFiber 5g6% sugar 30 g of 60% protein Vitamin A 2712IU54% Vitamin C 78 mg 95% 151 mg of calcium15% Iron 4 mg 22%

CHICKEN AND SHRIMP CURRY

Ingredients

- lbs. skinless chicken thighs, cut into small pieces 1 lb of shrimp

- Tbsp butter or coconut oil 1 cup chopped onion

- Tbsp curry powder 1 Tbsp cumin

- 1 Tbsp fennel seeds 2 tsp cardamom

- 1 Tbsp turmeric

- 1 cup canned coconut milk

- ¾ ketchup header

- salt and pepper to taste

Instructions

1.   Start by melting 5 Tbsp butter in a skillet over medium heat.

2.   Add chicken pieces and chopped onion with melted butter and pepper to taste. Bake for 5 to 8 min until chicken is cooked through.

3.   Add the curry powder, caraway, fennel seeds, cardamom, and turmeric. Bake for about 30 seconds until the spices are fragrant.

4.   Reduce the heat and add the tomato sauce and coconut milk. Stir to mix well.

5.   Mix shrimp, cover, and simmer for 5 to 8 min until shrimp is tender.

Prep time: 15 min; Servings: 8

Macros: Cal 323 Lipids 19g29% Saturated fat 11g55% Cholesterol 242 mg 81% Sodium 618 mg26% Potassium 517 mg 15% Total Carbs 8g3% 2g8% of dietary fiber 2 g of sugar 29 g58% protein Vitamin A6.5% Vitamin C9.1% Calcium 14% Iron 24.8%

KETO SEAFOOD dSOUP

Ingredients

- 1 lb of white fish, minced

- 10 to 12 shrimps, shelled and thawed

- 1 cup chopped crab meat

- 1 diced onion

- 2 garlic cloves, finely chopped

- 4 slices of bacon, cooked and sliced

- 1 radish daikon, peeled and chopped

- 2 cups fish broth or chicken

- 1 ½ cups whole coconut milk

- 2 Tbsp coconut oil

- Sea salt and freshly ground black pepper

Instructions

1.   Melt the coconut oil in a large saucepan over medium heat.

2. Add shrimp to pan and cook until pink, 2 to 3 minutes per side, set aside.

3. Add the onion and garlic for 3 to 4 minutes, stirring regularly.

4. Place the chopped daikon in the pan and cook for 4 to 5 min

5. Add fish and cook for 2 to 3 min, for the fish broth and stir, scratch the bottom of the pan.

6. Add the shrimp in the pan with the crabmeat, cover, and simmer for 12 to 15 min

7. For the coconut milk and season to taste.

8. Serve soup with sliced bacon.

Prep time: 6 min; Servings: 4

Macros: Protein 44 g / 32% Carbs 11 g / 8% Fat 36 g / 60%

KETO CALAMARI

Ingredients

- 1 lb of squid

- 3/4 cup coconut flour

- 1 egg

- ¼ cup sesame oil

- 2 Tbsp garlic powder

- 1 tsp ground cayenne pepper, optional

- 1 Tbsp onion powder

- 1 tsp salt

- 1 tsp pepper

- 1 cup sweet and spicy garlic and chili sauce

Instructions

1. Mix all dry ingredients in a large bowl. In a separate container. Beat the egg.

2.   Rinse the squid rings and tentacles and dry them with paper towels.

3.   Heat the sesame oil in a skillet over high heat. Make sure the oil covers the entire pan.

4.   Dip the pieces of squid in the egg and whisk the dry ingredients. Cook in oil for 2-3 min on each side and leave space between pieces of squid.

Prep time: 7 min; Servings: 2

Macros: Cal 581 | Carbs 7 g | Protein 24 g | Fat 28.4 g | Cholesterol 629 mg | Sodium 1268 mg | Fiber 6 g

BAKED HALIBUT WITH SOUR CREAM AND PARMESAN

Ingredients

- 2 halibut or other soft white fish, thawed when frozen and dried with paper towels

- salt and black pepper freshly ground to taste

- 3 Tbsp cream

- ¼ tsp garlic powder

- ¼ tsp dill (dried dill leaves)

- 2 Tbsp finely ground parmesan cheese

- 3 Tbsp sliced green onion (about 3 green onions)

Instructions

1   Thaw frozen halibut in a refrigerator overnight, place in a baking dish, and dry with a paper towel. Let the halibut come up to temperature while you prepare the other ingredients. Preheat oven to 375F / 190C.

2   Cut green onion; measure 2 Tbsp and chop finely. Keep the rest for garnish.

3   Mix of cream, garlic powder, and dill herbs in a small bowl. Add the finely grated parmesan and green onions. Spread over fish.

4   Cook the fish until the internal temperature reaches 145F / 62C.

Prep time:10 min; Servings: 2

GRILLED SCALLOPS WITH CREAM SAUCE

Ingredients

- 12 oz scallops

- 1 Tbsp avocado oil

- 2 tsp butter

- ½ cup thick whipped cream

- 1 Dijon mustard tsp (preferably whole wheat)

- ½ tsp fresh tarragon (or ¼ tsp dry)

- A pinch of of the salt sea (or to taste)

- Additional tarragon for garnish (optional)

Instructions

1. Rinse the scallops and dry thoroughly.

2. Heat a large skillet over medium heat. Add the avocado oil and then the butter.

3. Adding scallops to the pan and make sure they do not touch each other.

4. Cook the scallops for 3 to 5 min. Turn the scallops and brown them entirely on the other side. When the scallops are opaque, place them on a plate.

5. For the heavy cream, place the same pan over medium heat. Add the Dijon mustard and any liquid that has accumulated under the scallops. Bring the mixture to a boil and simmer until the sauce is thick enough to cover a spoon. Remove from heat and add tarragon and sea salt.

6. Serve the scallops with the sauce. Garnish with extra tarragon if desired.

Prep time:10 min; Servings: 6

Macros: Cal 282 Lipids 22 g Saturated fat 11 g 86 mg of cholesterol Sodium 272 mg 359 mg of Total potassium Carbs 4 g 1 g of Sugar 16 g 32% protein

WHITEFISH WITH PARMESAN AND PESTO

Ingredients

- 2 white fish fillets, about 6 oz each

- 3 Tbsp pine nuts

- 2 Tbsp parmesan

- ¼ tsp finely chopped garlic (1 garlic clove)

- 1 tsp basil pesto

- 1 ½ Tbsp mayonnaise

Instructions

1   Preheat the oven or toaster at 400°F / 200C. Spray individual pans with nonstick spray or olive oil (use a large saucepan if you do not have 1).

2   Remove fish from the refrigerator and let them reach the temperature while the oven is overheating. (It is essential to have the fish at room temperature. Otherwise, it will not be cooked until the lid is too brown).

3   Use a large chef's knife to finely chop the pine nuts and chop the garlic. Mix chopped pine nuts, parmesan cheese, chopped garlic, basil pesto, and mayonnaise.

4   Use a rubber scraper to spread the crust mixture evenly over the surface of each fish fillet. Apply it to the crust mixture.

5   Cooked fish for 10 to 15 min, until the fish is firm and the crust mixture begins to brown a little. (I cooked the fish pieces on the picture for 13 min). Serve hot.

Servings: 2; Prep time:30 min

WIRE CREAM AIL

Ingredients

- 1 Tbsp olive oil

- 1 lb (500 g) shrimp, with or without tail

- Salt and pepper to taste

- 2 Tbsp unsalted butter

- 6 garlic cloves, finely chopped

- ½ cup dry white wine or chicken broth

- 1 ½ cups of skimmed cream

- ½ cup grated fresh parmesan cheese

- 2 Tbsp chopped fresh parsley

Instructions

1   Heat the oil in a large skillet over medium heat. Season shrimp with salt and pepper and fry for 1-2 min per side until well cooked and pink. Transfer to a bowl; put aside.

2   Melt the butter in the same pan. Fry the garlic until fragrant (about 30 seconds). For the white wine or broth; reduce by half while scraping the lower parts of the pan.

3   Reduce heat to medium, add cream and simmer, stirring occasionally. Season with salt and pepper.

4   Add parmesan sauce and simmer for a minute until cheese melts and sauce thickens.

5   Add the shrimp in the pan, sprinkle with parsley.

Prep time: 10 min;

Macros: Cal 488 | Carbs 4 g | Protein 30 g | Fat 44 g Saturated Fat 25 g | Cholesterol 234 mg | Sodium 110 mg Potassium 223 mg | Vitamin A: 1765 IU | Vitamin C: 9.2 mg | Calcium: 375 mg | Iron: 2.8 mg

FILLET WITH GARLIC AND SHRIMP

Ingredients

- lean beef fillets or steak of your choice salt and pepper

- Tbsp olive oil 1 Tbsp butter

- 1 lb of shrimp, shelled and evaded 3 cloves of garlic, finely chopped

- Garlic butter:

- ¼ cup soft butter

- cloves of garlic, finely chopped 1 tsp chopped thyme

- 1 tsp minced rosemary 1 tsp minced oregano

Instructions

1   Place a medium skillet over high heat. Add olive oil and butter. Add the steaks. Cook on each side for 3 min or until golden brown.

2   Lower the temperature to medium to low. Cook the steaks. Remove and place on a plate.

3   Reduce the fire to a low. Add shrimp and garlic and cook for 2 to 3 minutes until they become opaque. Add the steaks back to the pan. Mix the butter, garlic, and chopped fresh herbs.

Prep time:5 min; Servings: 6

Macros: Cal 699 Lipids 32g49% Saturated fat 10 g 5g Carbs 1 g oFiber 1 g of sugar 94 g of protein

KETO TUNA MORNAY

Ingredients

- 1 batch of keto cheese sauce

- 400 g broccoli florets (14 oz)

- 425 g tuna, drained (15 oz)

- 100 g grated cheddar (4 oz)

Instructions

1   Preheat the oven to 180° C / 350° F.

2   Boil the broccoli until they are soft; do not boil them too much, as they will cook a bit more in the oven.

3   Place the broccoli in a baking dish evenly over the tuna. Pour the prepared cheese sauce and sprinkle with grated cheese.

4   Bake for 15-20 min until golden and bubbling. Let cool 5 min before serving.

Prep time:15 min; Servings: 4

Macros: Cal 632 | Carbs 9 g | Protein 34g | Fat 51 g | Fiber 2g | Sugar 1 g | Net Carbs 7 g

SHRIMP PAPER

Ingredients

- 2 lbs of shrimp, 907 g

- 16 cherry tomatoes, cut in half

- 2 small zucchini

- 1 yellow pepper, cut into pieces

- 2 Tbsp olive oil

- 2 crushed garlic cloves

- 1 tsp salt

- 1 tsp pepper

- 4 slices of lemon

- 1 Tbsp finely chopped parsley

Instructions

How to cook the pack of shrimp sheets on a grill

1   Prepare the shrimp and vegetables as follows and wrap the aluminum containers.

2   Bake shrimp paper packets for about 10 to 15 min on a hot grill or until vegetables are cooked through. Serve hot and sprinkle with parsley chopped and lemon juice.

Cooking with oven shrimp packages

1   Preheat oven to 400°F

2   Cut 4 large foil sheets, about 12-15 inches long.

3   Mix shrimp, tomatoes, and zucchini in olive oil, garlic, salt, and pepper and let stand in for 15 min and stir again.

4   Divide the shrimp and vegetable mixture over the pieces of aluminum and cover with a slice of lemon.

5   Fold aluminum wrappers over shrimps and vegetables to cover the food completely, then fold up and down to close.

6   Bake 15 to 20 min or until vegetables and shrimp are cooked through.

7   Serve hot and sprinkle with parsley chopped and lemon juice.

Prep time:10 min; Servings: 4

Macros: Cal 326 10 g oFat Saturated fat 1 g 8g Carbs 1 g oFiber 3 g of sugar 48 g of protein

ATLANTIC COD WITH HERB BUTTER AND HERBS

Ingredients

- 6 Tbsp unsalted butter, sweet

- 1/ 2 tsp garlic, finely chopped

- 1 tsp fresh parsley, finely chopped

- 1 tsp fresh thyme leaves

- tsp fresh basil, finely chopped

- ¼ tsp sea salt

- Tbsp extra virgin olive oil

- 6 Atlantic cod fillets of 4 oz

- Sea salt and black pepper to taste

- Fresh parsley, chopped, to decorate

Instructions

1.   Prepare garlic and herb butter by all ingredients in a medium bowl. Stir until garlic, herbs, and salt are evenly distributed over the soft butter.

2.   Transfer the butter mixture to the center of a plastic sheet and form a stem. Wrap them up in the refrigerator for 15 to 20 minutes to make them firm.

3.   Heat the olive oil in a skillet over medium heat. Dry the cod fillets with paper towels and season with salt and black pepper.

4.   Add the steaks to skillet and cook for 2 to 3 min or until golden brown. Cover each steak with an equal amount of herb butter and another 3-4 min While cooking, place the butter on the fillets as it melts.

5.   Remove from heat and transfer to individual dishes for serving. Sprinkle with melted herb butter and garnish with fresh chopped parsley, if desired.

Prep time:5 min; Servings: 6

Macros: Total Carbs 0.43 g Fiber 0.1 g Net Carbs 0.33 g Protein 43% Fat content: 56% Carbs 1%

HEALTHY OKRA SEAFOOD

Ingredients

- ½ cup cassava flour

- ⅓ cup speech juice

- ½ cup chopped celery

- 1 cup chopped onion

- 1 cup green pepper, seeded and minced

- 1 clove garlic, minced

- ½ lb sliced chicken and apple sausage

- 4 cups beef broth

- 2 cups of water

- 1 Tbsp coconut amino acids

- 1 ½ - 2 tsp salt

- 1 Tbsp Louisiana hot sauce

- 1 tsp Cajun spice blend

- 2 bay leaves

- ¼ tsp dried thyme leaves

- 1 can (14.5 g) diced tomatoes in juice

- 2 tsp divided gumbo-lime powder, optional

- 1 Tbsp avocado oil or more fat bacon

- 1 pack of 10 g oFrozen frost frozen okra

- 1 Tbsp white vinegar

- 8 g of drained crabmeat

- 1 ½ lbs medium uncooked shrimp, shelled and thawed

- Fresh parsley, minced, optional

Instructions

1   Heat ⅓ cup bacon in a large Dutch oven over medium heat. Sprinkle with cassava, and a smooth dough

appears. Cook this mixture, stirring almost constantly, for about 30 min, or until it turns to deep amber color. Do not let it burn; make this process happen slowly and gradually.

2   Add celery, onion, pepper, and garlic to a food processor and press several times until the mixture is finely chopped.

3   When the roux has a vibrant amber color, add the mixture of celery, onion, pepper, and garlic; Add the sliced sausage. Mix well, then add 1 cup water and beat well. Bring the mixture to a boil over medium heat

and cook for about 15 min. If necessary, add the second cup of water to prevent the dough from sticking to the bottom of the Dutch oven.

4   Meanwhile, boil 4 cups of beef broth in a medium-sized saucepan. Add the coconut amino acids, salt, hot sauce, Cajun spices, bay leaves, dried thyme, and diced tomatoes. Simmer for 2 hours over medium heat. If you have a gumbo girl add 1 tsp to the soup after 1 hour.

5   Meanwhile, heat 1 Tbsp avocado oil in the saucepan used to heat the beef broth. Add the thawed okra and vinegar and cook on medium heat for 15 min or until they are sticky and soft. Stir the okra with crabmeat and shrimp. Simmer for 45 minutes over low heat. If you have a fillet of okra, add the remaining tsp just before serving.

Servings: 6; Prep time:45 min

Macros: Cal 273 Lipids 13g20% Saturated fat 4 g Carbs 12g4% 2g8% oFiber 3g3% sugar 24 g48% protein

FRIED SALMON WITH CREAMY SAUCE

Ingredients

- pieces of salmon (about 4 g each)

- 1 Tbsp chopped fresh dill

- Olive oil

- Salt and pepper to taste For the sauce:

- 1 Tbsp chopped fresh dill

- ⅓ cup sour cream

- Tbsp mayonnaise

- 1 tsp Dijon mustard

- 1 Tbsp chopped capers

- ½ lemon juice and zest

- Salt and pepper to taste

Instructions

1   Make the sauce by mixing all the ingredients in a bowl; leave at room temperature while you prepare the salmon.

2   Preheat the oven to 400°F.

3   Place the salmon on a baking sheet lined with foil. Brush each piece with olive oil. Sprinkle with salt, pepper, and dill.

4   Bake 10 min.

5   Increase the temperature to 450°F and cook another 5-8 min.

6   Serve with a spoonful of sauce and garnish with dill and capers.

Prep time:5 min; Servings: 6

Macros: Cal 348 Lipids 27g Saturated fat 2g Carbs 1g 27 g protein

KETO CAJUN TRINITY

Ingredients

- 2 tsp

- 1 full celery, finely chopped

- ½ cup chopped mixed pepper

- 1 shallot

- 2 garlic cloves, finely chopped

- sea salt and black pepper, to taste

- 1 large egg

- 2 Tbsp mayonnaise

- 1 Tbsp Worcestershire sauce

- 1 tsp spicy brown mustard

- 1 tsp hot sauce

- ½ cup grated Parmesan cheese

- ½ cup crushed pork rind

- 1 lb of crab meat in pieces, without shell

- 2 Tbsp olive oil

Instructions

1.   Heat to the frying pan over medium heat. Heat the butter in the pan and add celery, pepper, shallots, garlic, sea salt, and black pepper. Bake until vegetables is transparent and soft, about 10 min

2.   Mix the egg, mayonnaise, Worcestershire, spicy brown mustard, and spicy sauce in a large bowl. Add the baked vegetables, and all ingredients are well absorbed. Mix the Parmesan and the pork rind. Fold the crab into the mixture.

3.   Cover a large baking sheet with parchment paper. Form the crab mixture into 8 patties. Place the patties on the prepared baking sheet and refrigerate for 1 to 2 hours.

4.   Cooked in olive oil in a large skillet over medium heat until crab cakes on both sides are golden and crisp.

Prep time:15 min; Servings: 2

Macros: Cal 412 Fat 28 g Carbs 4 g Fiber 1 g

CREAMY KETO SHRIMP WITH MEDITERRANEAN ZOODLES

Ingredients

- 2 zucchini medium size, spiralized

- 1 lb of shrimp, uncooked, deveined and without tail

- 1.5 Tbsp tomato puree

- 4 oz cream cheese

- ½ cup half and half

- 2 Tbsp thyme

- 2 Tbsp garlic powder

- 2 oregano Tbsp

- 1 Tbsp parsley flakes

- 1 Tbsp onion powder

- 1 tsp turmeric

- 1 Tbsp red pepper flakes

- ½ cup grated Parmesan cheese

Instructions

1.   Preheat the oven to 400° F. Melt butter in a cast iron skillet and add zoodles and shrimp.

2.   Mix the herbs, cream cheese, butter, and half and half in a small saucepan over medium heat. Stir regularly.

3.   Cook the noodles and shrimp for 5-8 min Remove the sauce and add it to shrimp and zoodles. Stir, add Parmesan cheese, and cook another 10 min.

Prep time:10 min; Servings: 4

Macros: Cal 381 | Carbs 8 g | Protein 31.8 g | Fat 21.9 g | Saturated Fat 12.8 g | Sodium 434 mg Fiber 4.2 g

GARLIC SQUID

Ingredients

- 10oz / 300g Squid

- ½ lemon juice

- 2 Tbsp olive oil

- 2 cloves garlic

- ⅓ cup boneless olives

- ½ cup arugula

- 2 Tbsp tomato puree

- 1 Tbsp dried basil

- ground pepper

- Parmesan cheese

Instructions

1   Cook the squid in a saucepan with a little water for 3-4 min, covered with a lid. Make sure the squid

is ready. Remove the extra water and add the lemon juice and olive oil.

2   Add the tomato puree and add 2 Tbsp water if necessary. Squeeze the garlic, add the dried basil and cracked pepper.

3   Garnish with parmesan or add another type of cheese.

KETO SHRIMP FAJITAS

Ingredients

- 1.5 lbs Fresh shrimp

- 1 large yellow pepper, finely sliced

- 1 medium green pepper, sliced thinly

- small red peppers sliced thinly

- 1 little chili, cut into thin slices

- medium red onions sliced thinly

- jalapenos in thin slices

- 3/4 cup finely chopped celery stalks Adobo (divided):

- 3 Lime gold lime, juice extract

- ¼ tsp garlic powder

- ½ tsp chili powder

- ½ tsp Spanish pepper

- ¼ tsp ground cumin

- ⅓ cup olive oil

- Salt and black pepper ground to taste

Instructions

1   Wash the shrimp thoroughly with water. Remove the bowl, head, and vein. Keep the tails intact. Dry with paper towels. Put aside.

2   In a bowl, mix olive oil, gold lime juice, garlic powder, chili powder, Spanish pepper, cumin, salt, and black pepper.

3   Pour marinade over the pepper and shrimp slices. Marinate for at least 15 min

4   Spread pepper, jalapeño pepper, celery, and half of the red onions in a baking dish and sprinkle with marinade. Bake at 400° F for 5 min.

5   Add the shrimp to the dish. Bake for 5 to 8 min..

6   Heat tortillas.

7   Serve with avocado slices and sour cream on the side.

Prep time:20 min; Servings: 8

Macros: Cal 158 | Carbs 5 g | Protein 13 g | Fat 10 g Saturated Fat 1 g | Polyunsaturated Fat 1 g | Monounsaturated Fat 7 g | Cholesterol 101 mg | Sodium 85 mg Potassium 290 mg | Fiber 3g | Sugar 1 g | Vitamin A: 650 IU | Vitamin C: 82.5 mg | Calcium: 50 mg | Iron: 0.9 mg

SHRIMP ALLA VODKA

Ingredients

- 1 lb of raw shrimp, shelled and sliced

- 4 g oFinely sliced prosciutto, diced

- Box of 28 g of organic crushed tomatoes (no added salt / low-carb)

- 15 oz organic diced tomatoes (no added salt / low Carbs)

- 1 cup thick whipped cream

- ⅓ cup vodka (without taste)

- 5 fresh basil leaves

- 2 garlic cloves, finely chopped

- 1 Tbsp olive oil

- A pinch of salt and pepper

- Parmesan grated to cover

- zucchini, spiral "spaghetti" about ½ per person

Instructions

1.   Heat a large skillet over medium heat, add olive oil and ham. Fry the bacon for 2 min and add garlic to cook for another minute. Be careful not to brown the garlic. Remove from heat and scrape all browned parts of the bottom of the pan.

2.   Slowly reduce vodka, then add tomato sauce, dried basil, parsley, heavy cream, salt, and pepper. Cook over medium heat with lid overstuffed for 25 min, stirring occasionally.

3.   While the sauce is boiling, you can prepare your zucchini noodles or "zoodles." Cut each end of the zucchini and spiralize. Cut into traditional spaghetti pieces and set aside.

4.   After boiling for 25 min, add the sauce and cook another 5 min

5.   Add zucchini noodles to your plate, top with shrimp and grated parmesan cheese. Garnish with fresh basil leaves.

Prep time: 5 min; Servings: 2

Macros: Cal212 Lipids 11g17% Saturated fat 8g50% Carbs 7g2% 2g8% oFiber 3g3% sugar 12 g of 24% protein

CRAB OMELET WITH AVOCADO AND HERBS

Ingredients

- 3 eggs

- 1 tsp chopped parsley

- 1 tsp chopped chives

- ½ tsp sea salt or kosher

- ½ tsp ground black pepper

- 1 Tbsp butter

- ½ oz grated Parmesan about 2 Tbsp

- 2 oz crab meat into about ½ cup pieces

- 1 green onion, finely sliced

- ½ sliced avocado

- 1 Tbsp sour cream

Instructions

1. Break the eggs in a small bowl. Add the onions, parsley, salt, and pepper

2.   Place a 10-inch nonstick skillet over medium heat, add the butter, and stir until it melts.

3.   Pour the beaten eggs in the pan. Shake the pan to cover the bottom of the pan. Fry the eggs over medium heat until the edges are firm, and the medium is barely cooked for 3-4 min Deflate the big bubbles with the teeth of a fork.

4.   Sprinkle half of the Parmesan on half of the tortilla. Cover the crabmeat with cheese and green onions. Place the avocado on the green onions and cover with remaining Parmesan cheese.

5.   Using a spatula, fold the empty half of the eggs to form a semicircle. Remove from heat and transfer to a plate. Sprinkle with fresh herbs to taste and decorate with a Tbsp sour cream. Serve immediately.

Prep time:10 min; Servings: 1

Macros: Cal 557 (28%).

SALMON BROCCOLI FUN BAG

Ingredients

- ½ cup broccoli, minced

- 1 celery stalk, finely chopped

- ¼ leek, cut, clean and cut

- A pinch of chopped fresh rosemary, chili powder, and curry powder

- Cayenne pepper to taste (optional)

- g of wild salmon

- ¼ sliced avocado

- Coriander, sliced green onions and sliced watermelon radish to taste

- 1-2 Tbsp cerebral octane oil

- Cooked and cooled white rice (optional), flavored with ground turmeric

Instructions

4.   Cook the salmon using your preferred method (poaching is recommended).

5.   While the salmon cooks, prepare the base of the leek with broccoli. Generously season a pot of water with salt and boil. Add broccoli, celery, and leek and cook 10 min or until tender.

6.   Drain the vegetables and save about ½ cup the cooking liquid.

7.   Transfer the vegetables to a blender and mix until puree, add a Tbsp boiling water at a time until it reaches a consistency of the vegetable puree. (You can also do it in your pot with a hand blender). Add rosemary, chili powder, curry powder, and cayenne pepper (if used) and mix well.

8.   Put the broccoli leek base in a bowl and cover with rice, cooked salmon, avocado, and remaining vegetables. Spray with cerebral octane oil and serve hot.

Prep time:20 min; Servings: 1

Macros: Cal 374 Fat 20.4 g Carbs 14 g Fiber 6.3 g Protein 26.6 g Carbs 7.7 g

SALMON WITH TOMATO AND CUCUMBER

Ingredients

- 5 oz wild salmon fillets, skinless

- 1 ball oFennel, thickly sliced

- 1 large cucumber

- ½ cup boneless green olives

- 3 Tbsp butter or herb butter

- Fresh thyme leaves

- 2 extra virgin olive oil Tbsp

Instructions

1. Preheat the oven to 350° F.

2. Place the salmon on the fennel and the dotted ghee on the salmon. Sprinkle fresh thyme leaves on top.

3. Bake the salmon in the oven for 15 min

4. While the salmon is in the oven, twist the cucumber into noodles and allow the excess water to drain by pressing gently.

5. Put the noodles in a bowl and dress them with extra virgin olive oil.

6. Remove the salmon from the oven.

7. Put the noodles on a plate and put the salmon on it. Add the green olives and sprinkle with salt to taste.

Prep time:10 min; Servings: 2

Macros: Cal 502.4 Protein 38.9 g Carbs 15.6 g Fiber 5.32 g Carbs 8.6 g Sugar 7.1 g Fat 31.6 g Saturated Fat 4.38 g

TANDOORI OVEN SALMON

Ingredients

- 4 oz wild salmon fillets

- g of unsweetened natural coconut milk yogurt

- 1 Tbsp raw apple cider vinegar

- 1 Tbsp avocado oil

- 1 tsp ground ginger or 1 inch fresh ginger mixed

- 1 tsp ground turmeric

- 1 tsp green cardamom seeds

- 1 tsp Ceylon cinnamon

- 1 tsp cloves

- 1 tsp cumin seeds

Instructions

1.   Prepare the tandoori salmon. Mix the coconut yogurt in a bowl with all the herbs. Put the salmon in the pan and cover. Leave to marinate for 30 min (either at the counter if you plan to cook immediately, or in the fridge if you plan to cook later).

2.   Preheat the oven to 350° F. Cover a baking sheet with aluminum foil.

3.   Remove the salmon from the marinade and place the skin on the baking sheet.

4.   Bake for 5 min Lift the oven rack and grill the salmon for 2-3 min until a light brown crust appears.

Prep time:15 min; Servings: 2

Macros: Cal 432 Protein 34 g Carbs 22.1 g Fiber 8.2 g Sugar 7.8 g Carbs

13.9 g Fat 23 g Saturated Fat 10 g

WILD SALMON OVEN WITH ASPARAGUS AND FENNEL

Ingredients

- 21 oz wild salmon (keta/king/sockeye)

- cups of asparagus

- ½ cup fennel, cut into thin slices

- medium avocados

- 1 Tbsp coconut amino acids

- 1 Tbsp dried seaweed

- 1 tsp Himalayan pink salt

- 1 Tbsp fresh lemon juice

- 1 extra virgin olive oil Tbsp

- Fennel leaves

- Chili flakes (optional)

Instructions

1. Put the salmon in the large bowl, then add the ingredients for the marinade. Amino coconut, dried seaweed, honey, salt, and lemon juice. Mix well and let stand for 20 min

2. Preheat the oven to 350° F.

3. Steamed asparagus and let them cool.

4. Put the sliced fennel in a heat-resistant pan and add the salmon

5. Place the baking sheet in the center of the oven and bake for about 10 min until it is cooked through.

6. Cut them in half and cut the avocados, place them on a plate or serving plate and transfer the salmon to the fennel.

7.   Sprinkle with extra virgin olive oil and garnish with fennel leaves, chili flakes, and Himalayan pink salt to taste.

Prep time: 15 min; Servings: 4

Macros: Cal 537.7 Protein 50.9 g Carbs 38.1 g Fiber 24.9g Sugar 11.9 g Fat

24.6 g Saturated Fat 1.55 g

KETO CEVICHE

Ingredients

- Fresh halibut from the wild, cubed (preferably sushi grade)

- 1 lime juice

- 2 brain octane oil tsp

- A pinch of Himalayan pink salt

- 1 small avocado, diced

- 1 organic green onion, thinly sliced

- 1 Tbsp chopped fresh organic coriander

- Optional: 2 Tbsp diced pickled radish

Instructions

1. Combine lime juice, brain octane oil, and salt in a medium bowl.

2.   Put the rest of the ingredients in the bowl and stir gently.

3.   Divide into 2 portions.

Prep time: 15 min Servings: 2

Macros: Cal 198 Protein 20 g Carbs 2 g Fiber 2 g Sugar 0 g Fat 10 g Saturated Fat 5 g

COD IN THE PAN

Ingredients

- 2 ½ lbs of cod fillets

- Tbsp unsalted butter, sliced

- seasoning

- ¼ tsp garlic powder

- ½ tsp table salt

- ¼ tsp ground pepper

- ¾ tsp ground pepper

- A few lemon slices

- Herbs, parsley or coriander

Instructions

1. Combine the herbal ingredients in a small bowl.

2. Cut the cord into small pieces, if desired. Season all sides of the cod with the herbs.

3.   Heat 2 Tbsp butter in a large skillet over medium-high heat. As soon as the butter melts, add the cod to the pan. Cook for 2 min

4.   Lower the heat to medium. Turn the cod over, cover with the rest of the butter and cook for another 3-4 min

5.   The butter melts completely, and the fish boils. (Do not overcook the cod, it will soften and collapse completely).

6.   Sprinkle the cod with fresh lemon juice. Cover with fresh herbs if desired. Serve immediately.

Prep time:5 min; Servings: 4

Macros: Cal 294 Fat 18 g Saturated fat 11 g Cholesterol 118 mg Sodium 385 mg Potassium 712 mg Protein 30 g

LEMON FISH CAKE WITH AVOCADO SAUCE

Ingredients

- 1 lb of boneless raw fish (preferably local and game)

- ¼ cup coriander (leaves and stems)

- Pinch of salt

- A pinch of chili flakes

- 1-2 garlic cloves (optional)

- 1-2 Tbsp coconut oil or butter fed on frying grass

- Neutral oil to grease your hands, like avocado oil

- 2 ripe avocados

- 1 lemon, juiced

- Pinch of salt

- 2 Tbsp water

Instructions

1.	In a food processor, add the fish, herbs, garlic (if used), salt, chili, and fish. Blitz until everything is evenly combined.

2.	In a large skillet over medium heat, add the coconut oil or butter and stir to cover.

3.	Oil your hands and roll the fish mixture into 6 patties.

4.	Add cakes to the hot pan. Cook on both sides until golden and cooked through.

5.   While the fish cakes are cooked, add all the ingredients for the dipping sauce (from the lemon juice) in a small food processor or blender and mix until the dough is smooth and creamy. Try the mixture and add more lemon juice or salt if necessary.

6.   When the fish cakes are cooked, serve them hot with a dipping sauce.

Servings: 6; Prep time:15 min

Macros: Cal 69 Fat 6.5 g Saturated Fat 1.9 g Cholesterol 6 mg Sodium 54 mg Total Carbs 2.7 g Fiber 2.1g Sugar 0.2 g Carbs 0.6 g Protein 1.1 g

TOMATO BROTH COD POACHED

Ingredients

- 1 lb wild-caught cod fillet, cut into 3-inch squares

- A 28 oz can of organic peeled whole tomatoes (BPA free), drained

- 1.5 cups pastured chicken broth

- pinch of saffron (about 15 threads)

- 2 bay leaves

- 3 avocado oil Tbsp

- Sea salt to taste

Instructions

1.   Add the oil to a pan over medium heat. Put the peeled tomatoes in the pan with your hands. Add broth, saffron, bay leaf, and salt to taste.

2.   Bring the broth over low heat over medium heat and reduce the heat.

3.   Add the cod fillets and cover, simmer for 5-7 min, or only until the fish begins to crumble.

4.   Serve the fish with tomato broth.

Servings: 2 Prep time: 20 min

Macros: Cal 167 Fat 10.3 g Saturated Fat 1 g Cholesterol 35 mg Sodium 100 mg Total Carbs 1.6 g Dietary Fiber 0.4 g Sugar 0 g Protein 18 g Calcium: 7 mg Potassium 65 mg

KETO FISH AND CHIPS

Ingredients

- 250 g firm white fish, preferably cod

- ⅓ cup sour cream

- tsp apple cider vinegar

- cloves of garlic passed through a press

- Kosher salt to taste

- ½ cup whey protein isolate

- 1 tsp of baking powder

- ¼ tsp garlic powder

- 1 / 4-1 / 2 tsp kosher salt to taste

- 1 egg

- 1 Tbsp sour cream or coconut cream

- 2 tsp apple cider vinegar

- coconut oil or cooking oil of your choice

- 1 batch oFries with 8 jicama tortillas

- 1 bunch of our keto mayonnaise

- lemon

- vinegar

Instructions

1. Mix sour cream (or coconut), vinegar, garlic, and season with salt. Cut the fish through the meat grain into strips about 2.5 cm wide and add them to the cream marinade. Treat and allow to cool for 2 hours, preferably overnight.

2. Prepare your frying station by adding enough oil to a skillet or saucepan to be about ½ inch deep. You can save a lot oFat by using a narrower pan and frying them in batches. Heat the oil over medium / low heat while stirring the fish.

3. Combine whey protein, baking powder, garlic powder, and salt in a shallow dish or dish. Beat the egg in a second dish or a plate with cream and vinegar.

4. Cover the fish by lightly removing the excess marinade, dipping in the egg mixture, followed by the whey protein mixture, immediately putting it in hot oil and directly spraying the top. You want to cook the fish quickly after cooking to get the best sharpness. Cook on both sides

until golden and place on a paper-covered plate for a few min

5. Serve immediately on a bed of potato chips with jicama, lots of lemons, mayonnaise and a pinch of vinegar.

Prep time: 20 min; Servings: 6

Macros: Cal 242 Fat 13 g Saturated fat 6 g Cholesterol 158 mg Sodium 427

mg Potassium 802 mg Carbs 1 g Sugar 1 g Protein 26 g